Elements of Mental Illness
Mental Health Has Many Versions
Your 12th Psychiatric Consultation.
William Yee M.D., J.D.
Copyright Applied for

Prologue

Having practiced psychiatry without
interruption since 1972 in Michigan,
Indiana, Kentucky, California, and Texas.
I have struggled with the concepts of
mental health and mental illness for fifty
one years.

The reader should understand that this
book's primary focus is an introduction to
the landscape of mental illness and
interventions with medications.

The intention is to introduce the patient
and student to the broad outline of the
diagnosis and symptoms of mental illness.
The intent is to introduce the patient to
the treatment of mental illness with a few
specific medications explored in detail to
illustrate the strategy of adding
medications to healthy living and other
treatments of mental illness.

1 of 64

The patient is the most important part of the treatment team.
The patient should eventually know more about his mental illness than the psychiatrist.

First, the patient has a unique version of his mental illness that no one else has. He experiences his mental illness throughout the day every day.

The psychiatrist only has an occasional biopsy of the patient's mental illness and will never know the breadth and depth and details of the mental illness as well as the patient.

Second, the patient must study only his mental illness while the psychiatrist must study all mental illness and all medical conditions that intersect mental illness.

Nobody can know everything and keep up with the myriad daily advances of all mental illness and all medical problems as they intersect mental illnesses.

The patient can survey the internet daily for advances in his mental illness and his medications.

2 of 64

After a time, the patient should know his mental illness and his medications better than the psychiatrist.

That only happens in a perfect world.

However, I have met diligent patients that have educated me about their mental illness and medications and enjoyed working with them.

On average, these patients fare better than the rest of my patients.

There are many versions of mental illness. One version allows for many genders. In fact, our national version allows an individual to create a personal gender daily, and then change their personal version daily.

Another version makes homosexuality a mental illness.

Another version makes homosexuality a capital crime subject to the death penalty.

Beheading in public is videotaped and posted on the internet by some foreign governments.

Mental illness is subject to political and cultural definitions outside the scope of science.

At the end of the day, everyone has their own version of mental illness.

It is necessary to find out what that person views as mental illness before attempting to treat the mental illness.

Mental health has the same pattern. Every culture has an ideal norm that is presented to children as the goal in life.

Each family has their own version of that cultural norm of mental health.
Each person in the family has their own version of the cultural norm of mental health.

The version is shaped by age, place in the sibship, health, intellect, economic context, social context, community context, etc.

Medicine is a scientific discipline with an ethical basis, do no harm, primum non nocere, non-maleficence, act only if the benefit is greater than the harm.

4 of 64

This is a special case of the Golden Rule, do unto others as you would have them do unto you.

The diagnosis of mental illness is shaped by culture, politics, and money. This distorts the scientific method.

The current practice is to collect symptoms and run them through a mathematical model such as factor analysis to discover mental illness.

This is science in the sense that it identifies clusters of symptoms that can be researched for underlying mental illness.

However, these collections of symptoms are used to determine if psychiatric treatment will be a benefit of an insurance policy, or a basis for disability, or a basis for the insanity defense, or a basis for assigning a conservator, or a basis for loss of legal rights. All of these are political, cultural and economic activities that are outside the scope of science and can in fact distort science and scientific research.

The distortion of science and scientific research is most easily seen in the pharmaceutical marketing of thalidomide and opiates, and the civil litigation over cigarettes and health, and the civil litigation over asbestos and health, and the marketing of sugar and research into heart disease.

The above marketing and civil litigation are showcases for how money corrupts the government and the judiciary.

Because the diagnostic categories are vague, based upon science distorted by money and politics, what should the psychiatrist and the patient do?

Most seasoned psychiatrists treat symptoms and use diagnosis only for the purpose of submitting bills to insurance companies, completing disability forms, or testifying in court regarding issues of competency, or insanity.

Before we proceed, I should advise the reader that diligence in the practice of:
1. Dietary hygiene,
2. Sleep hygiene.
3. Physical hygiene and exercise.

6 of 64

4. Mental hygiene including meditation.
5. Social hygiene including the Golden Rule.

will do more for the reader than any treatment or medication that I can offer.

Diligence in the practice of good hygiene will improve physical and mental health and avoid anxiety, depression, and disease.

The reader should investigate the above hygiene as part of healthy living to avoid the need for psychiatric treatment.

When the population is graphed on the X axis of the X, Y graph, a bell shape curve is created.

```
|                    **
|                   ***
|                  *****
|                 *******
|               **************
|              ******************
|            ************************
|          ****************************
|0***1***2***3***4***5***6***7**8***9***10
```

The horizontal is the severity of symptoms.

The vertical is the percentage of patients afflicted with that severity of symptom.

At the left end of the graph is the lowest severity and at the right end is the highest severity of symptoms on a scale of 0 to 10.

Anxiety, depression, hallucinations, delusions, paranoia, and other symptoms can be rated on a scale of 0 to 10. 0 is none and 10 is the worst that the patient has ever experienced.

Mental illness and disability afflict the five percent of the population at the right end of the graph.

Most people have occasional symptoms without mental illness throughout their lives.

Psychiatrists are expensive and insurance and health care facilities usually confine psychiatrists to prescribing psychotropic medications. Psychiatrists are basically pill mills.

Psychotherapies such as DBT-Dialectic Behavior Therapy, CBT - Cognitive

Behavior Therapy, EMDR-Eye Movement Desensitizaton Therapy, Desensitization Therapy, Flooding Therapy, indvidual, group, and family therapies are relegated to psychologists, social workers, psychiatric technicians and other mental health workers.

The reader should study the relationship between Hellen Keller and Anne Sullivan to understand the potential of psychotherapy without psychotropic medications. This is very intensive, extensive, and expensive treatment with great potential. Perhaps with the development of Artificial Intelligence and robotics it will eventually become available.

Artificial Intelligence and robotics may eventually offer effective cures for schizophrenia, autism, personality disorders, and behavior disorders that are currently refractory to psychiatric interventions. Time will tell.

Schizophrenia includes but is not limited to the following symptoms:
Hallucinations   0 1 2 3 4 5 6 7 8 9 10
9 of 64

Delusions   0 1 2 3 4 5 6 7 8 9 10
Paranoia   0 1 2 3 4 5 6 7 8 9 10
Blocked Thoughts   0 1 2 3 4 5 6 7 8 9 10
Disorganized (word salad a 10)
   Thoughts   0 1 2 3 4 5 6 7 8 9 10
   Behaviors   0 1 2 3 4 5 6 7 8 9 10
    Hygiene   0 1 2 3 4 5 6 7 8 9 10
    Dress   0 1 2 3 4 5 6 7 8 9 10
    Etiquette   0 1 2 3 4 5 6 7 8 9 10
    Boundaries   0 1 2 3 4 5 6 7 8 9 10
    Legal   0 1 2 3 4 5 6 7 8 9 10
    Health   0 1 2 3 4 5 6 7 8 9 10
    Homeless   0 1 2 3 4 5 6 7 8 9 10
    Friendless   0 1 2 3 4 5 6 7 8 9 10
   Affect   0 1 2 3 4 5 6 7 8 9 10
    Flat   0 1 2 3 4 5 6 7 8 9 10
    Odd   0 1 2 3 4 5 6 7 8 9 10
    Autistic   0 1 2 3 4 5 6 7 8 9 10

Bipolar Disorder includes but is not
limited to the following symptoms:
Mood swings   0 1 2 3 4 5 6 7 8 9 10
   Rapid   0 1 2 3 4 5 6 7 8 9 10
Affect   0 1 2 3 4 5 6 7 8 9 10
   Depressed   0 1 2 3 4 5 6 7 8 9 10
   Manic   0 1 2 3 4 5 6 7 8 9 10
Hallucinations   0 1 2 3 4 5 6 7 8 9 10
Delusions   0 1 2 3 4 5 6 7 8 9 10
Paranoia   0 1 2 3 4 5 6 7 8 9 10

10 of 64

Disorganized (flight of ideas a 10)
    Thoughts   0 1 2 3 4 5 6 7 8 9 10
    Racing   0 1 2 3 4 5 6 7 8 9 10
Suicidal thoughts   0 1 2 3 4 5 6 7 8 9 10
Homicidal thoughts   0 1 2 3 4 5 6 7 8 9 10
    Behaviors   0 1 2 3 4 5 6 7 8 9 10
    Hygiene   0 1 2 3 4 5 6 7 8 9 10
    Dress   0 1 2 3 4 5 6 7 8 9 10
    Etiquette   0 1 2 3 4 5 6 7 8 9 10
    Boundary   0 1 2 3 4 5 6 7 8 9 10
    Legal   0 1 2 3 4 5 6 7 8 9 10
    Health   0 1 2 3 4 5 6 7 8 9 10
    Homeless   0 1 2 3 4 5 6 7 8 9 10
    Friendless   0 1 2 3 4 5 6 7 8 9 10
    Gambling   0 1 2 3 4 5 6 7 8 9 10
    Hypergraphia   0 1 2 3 4 5 6 7 8 9 10
    Speech   0 1 2 3 4 5 6 7 8 9 10
    Hypersexuality   0 1 2 3 4 5 6 7 8 9 10
    Credit spending   0 1 2 3 4 5 6 7 8 9 10
    Risky Behaviors   0 1 2 3 4 5 6 7 8 9 10

Depression includes but is not limited to
the following symptoms:
Depressed feelings   0 1 2 3 4 5 6 7 8 9 10
Hopelessness   0 1 2 3 4 5 6 7 8 9 10
Guilt   0 1 2 3 4 5 6 7 8 9 10
Low self esteem   0 1 2 3 4 5 6 7 8 9 10
Worthlessness   0 1 2 3 4 5 6 7 8 9 10
Poverty of thought   0 1 2 3 4 5 6 7 8 9 10
Anergy   0 1 2 3 4 5 6 7 8 9 10
11 of 64

Motor Deceleration	0 1 2 3 4 5 6 7 8 9 10
Slowed thoughts	0 1 2 3 4 5 6 7 8 9 10
Hypersomnia	0 1 2 3 4 5 6 7 8 9 10
Hyposomnia	0 1 2 3 4 5 6 7 8 9 10
Agitation	0 1 2 3 4 5 6 7 8 9 10
Suicidal thoughts	0 1 2 3 4 5 6 7 8 9 10
Homicidal thoughts	0 1 2 3 4 5 6 7 8 9 10

Suicidal and homicidal thoughts and impulses tend to occur together.

That is why there are so many newspaper stories about suicide and homicide. A person will kill their spouse, their attorney, their doctor, their parent, their child, and then commit suicide on the spot.

That is why many mass murderers will end a killing spree with their own suicide, or suicide by cop.

I had patients tell me they went into the psychiatrist's office with the intent of committing suicide in front of the psychiatrist, then at the last second decided to shoot the psychiatrist instead.

Anxiety includes but is not limited to:

Anxious feelings	0 1 2 3 4 5 6 7 8 9 10
Panic attacks	0 1 2 3 4 5 6 7 8 9 10
Fast heart rate	0 1 2 3 4 5 6 7 8 9 10
Pounding heart	0 1 2 3 4 5 6 7 8 9 10
Sweating	0 1 2 3 4 5 6 7 8 9 10
Shakes	0 1 2 3 4 5 6 7 8 9 10
Nightmares	0 1 2 3 4 5 6 7 8 9 10
Flashbacks	0 1 2 3 4 5 6 7 8 9 10
Specific Phobias	0 1 2 3 4 5 6 7 8 9 10
Generalized anxiety	0 1 2 3 4 5 6 7 8 9 10
Obsessions	0 1 2 3 4 5 6 7 8 9 10
Compulsions	0 1 2 3 4 5 6 7 8 9 10
Avoidance	0 1 2 3 4 5 6 7 8 9 10
Dependency	0 1 2 3 4 5 6 7 8 9 10

There are thought disorders:
Body Dysmorphic
Disorder   0 1 2 3 4 5 6 7 8 9 10

There are behavior disorders. The behavior disorders respond poorly to psychiatric interventions. At the end of the day a few patients control their behaviors. It is not known if the control is the result of treatment.

Behavior disorders include:

Bulimia	0 1 2 3 4 5 6 7 8 9 10
Anorexia	0 1 2 3 4 5 6 7 8 9 10

13 of 64

Conduct Disorder   0 1 2 3 4 5 6 7 8 9 10

The personality disorders can be viewed as behavior disorders with behaviors that are deeply engrained, fixed and refractory to treatment:

Cluster A (Strange) these personalities do not accept the cultural norms in thought and behaviors and include

Paranoid Personality Disorder: these personalities have pervasive paranoia that does not allow the person to engage in shared thoughts and activities due to an inability to trust.

Schizoid Personality Disorder: these personalities have pervasive odd thoughts and behaviors that do not allow the person to share activities based on empathy and emotional resonance.

Schizotypal PD these personalities have a pervasive autism without the capacity for shared emotional experiences and activities.

14 of 64

Cluster B (Predatory)

Antisocial Personality Disorder:
Antisocial personalities use physical
aggression and intellectual aggression
and do not allow laws to set boundaries
on their behaviors. They take without
giving and lack empathy or remorse.

Borderline Personality Disorder:
Borderline personalities often present as
predatory victims. They manipulate
others to aggression. They have numerous
short-term relationships that start with
an intense honeymoons and end in
equally intense and acrimonious
separations. They tend to burn out their
friends and relatives and end up alone
without a support system. They take
without giving. They lack empathy and
remorse and accuse others of abuse. They
blame others for their behaviors. Women's
prisons are notoriously difficult places to
work and many psychiatrists refuse to
work in women's prisons.

Borderline personalities present as a
particularly difficult group of patients in
the Department of State Hospitals-
Coalinga which is located at the edge of
15 of 64

the Coastal Mountain Range on the western side of Fresno County. This group is unique among all of the mental health facilities in the United States.

Histrionic Personality Disorder: Histrionic personalities have very intense emotional displays often with the object of seeking attention and or help.

Narcissistic Personality Disorder: Narcissistic Personalities are totally engrossed with themselves and little empathy or interest in the thoughts and feelings of others. Sharing and helping others is not one of their skill sets, or are shallow displays to disguise their exploitation of others.

Cluster C (Frightened)
Avoidant Personality Disorder: The avoidant personalities avoid engagement and activities.

Dependent Personality Disorder: The dependent personalities rely upon their parents to care for them and seek out others to care for them throughout their lives. They do not develop independent living skills and they do not care for others.

Obsessive-Compulsive Personality Disorder: The obsessive-compulsive personalities is consumed with obsessive thoughts and ritualistic behaviors.

The personality disorders do not seek to change themselves.

They focus on changing others. They rarely seek psychiatric treatment for the purpose of introspection and change. They are more often referred by family members than seeking treatment.

Specific Behavior Disorders include:

Trichotillomania: pulling eyelashes, eyebrows and hair off their bodies.

Motor Tics: Tourette's disorder is an example and manifests with a combination of vocal and motor movements that are abrupt, without thought, and may include potty mouth, or coprolalia, foul language and curses blurted out without thought or intention.

Bulimia: excessive eating. Psychiatric treatments often fail and surgery results. Bariatric Surgery is often employed when psychiatric treatment fails. Death and serious health problems can result from Bariatric Surgery. The failure rate for Bariatric Surgery is substantial.

Success of bariatric surgery is defined as loss of 50% of excess body weight. If you are two hundred pounds overweight, then one hundred pounds overweight is a success. There is a 15% failure rate within a year and a 30% failure rate after two years.

Bariatric surgery comes at a high cost, including but not limited to:
Acid reflux
Anesthesia-related risks
Chronic nausea and vomiting
Dilation of esophagus
Inability to eat certain foods
Infection
Obstruction of stomach
Weight gain or failure to lose weight
Dumping syndrome, a condition that can lead to symptoms like nausea and dizziness

Bleeding internally or profuse bleeding of themsurgical wound
Blood clots
Bowel obstruction
Breakage
Cardiac problems
Dumping syndrome
Gallstones
Hernias
Intestine perforation
Intestine ulceration
Iron deficiency
Leakage
Low blood sugar
Malnutrition
Obstruction of the pouch, anastomotic connection, or bowel obstruction
Pulmonary problems
Ulcers
Skin separation
Spleen and other organ injury
Stomach perforation
Stomach ulceration
Stricture
Vitamin deficiency
Vomiting and numerous other complications

Medications for Mood Disorders including Bipolar Disorder, Schizoaffective

Disorder and Mood Disorder NOS include primarily mood stabilizers and the antipsychotic medications.

Before medications are taken the patient should review the FDA Label for those medications.

Then review of information available on the internet for that medication as information will appear on the internet before it finds its way to the FDA label after the FDA's initial release for commercial marketing.

The following are lists of side effects for selected medications in the treatment of mental illness.

Mood stabilizers include:

1. lithium (Lithonate)
2. carbamazepine (Tegretol)
3. lamotrigine (Lamictal)
4. valproate (Depakote)

The mood stabilizers have serious side effects and it is very important to find the lowest effective dose and minimize the exposure to these medications.

20 of 64

Unfortunately, although lithium is the most effective mood stabilizer, it has been found to lose effect over time.

Side effects of lithium include but are not limited to:

1. The black box warning for lithium is Lithium toxicity is closely related to serum lithium levels, and can occur at doses close to therapeutic levels. This requires monitoring blood levels.
   The patient should be encouraged to drink on average 64 ounces of liquid daily to avoid dehydration.
2. Unmasking of Brugada Syndrome resulting in sudden death from cardiac complications associated with syncope or palpitations.
3. nephrogenic diabetes insipidus
4. polyuria
5. polydipsia
6. nephrotic syndrome
7. glomerular interstitial fibrosis
8. nephron atrophy
9. renal failure
10. encephalopathic syndrome with weakness, lethargy, fever, tremulousness and confusion,

extrapyramidal symptoms,
leukocytosis, elevated serum
enzymes, BUN, and FBS
11. fine hand tremor
12. mild thirst may occur during initial
therapy for the acute manic phase
and may persist throughout
treatment.
13. Transient and mild nausea and
general discomfort may also appear
during the first few days of lithium
administration.
14. Diarrhea
15. Vomiting
16. drowsiness,
17. muscular weakness
18. lack of coordination may be early
signs of lithium intoxication
19. Giddiness
20. Ataxia
21. blurred vision
22. Tinnitus
23. large output of dilute urine
24. Central Nervous System:
25. Tremor
26. muscle hyperirritability
27. Fasciculations
28. Twitching
29. clonic movements of whole limbs
30. Hypertonicity

31. Ataxia
32. choreoathetotic movements
33. hyperactive deep tendon reflex,
34. extrapyramidal symptoms including
35. acute dystonia
36. cogwheel rigidity
37. blackout spells
38. epileptiform Seizures
39. slurred speech
40. Dizziness
41. Vertigo
42. downbeat nystagmus
43. incontinence of urine or feces,
44. Somnolence
45. psychomotor retardation
46. Restlessness
47. Confusion
48. Stupor
49. Coma
50. tongue movements
51. tics,
52. Tinnitus
53. Hallucinations
54. poor memory
55. slowed intellectual functioning
56. startled response
57. worsening of organic brain syndromes
58. Pseudotumor cerebri
59. Papilledema

60. enlargement of the blind spot
61. constriction of visual fields
62. blindness
63. optic atrophy
64. Cardiovascular
65. cardiac arrhythmia,
66. Hypotension
67. peripheral circulatory collapse
68. Bradycardia
69. sinus node dysfunction
70. Anorexia
71. Nausea
72. Vomiting
73. Diarrhea
74. gastritis,
75. salivary gland swelling
76. abdominal pain
77. excessive salivation
78. Flatulence
79. indigestion
80. Glycosuria
81. decreased creatinine clearance
82. Albuminuria
83. oliguria,
84. drying and thinning of hair
85. alopecia,
86. anesthesia of skin
87. Acne
88. chronic folliculitis
89. xerosis cutis
90. psoriasis or its exacerbation

91. Generalized pruritus with
92. Rash
93. cutaneous ulcers
94. angioedema
95. blurred vision
96. dry mouth
97. Impotence
98. sexual dysfunction
99. euthyroid goiter and/or
100. hypothyroidism
101. Myxedema
102. Low T3 and T4.
103. Iodine uptake may be elevated
104. Hyperthyroidism
105. EEG
106. diffuse slowing
107. widening of frequency spectrum
108. potentiation and disorganization of background rhythm.
109. EKG Changes
110. reversible flattening
111. isoelectricity
112. inversion of T-waves.
113. Fatigue
114. Lethargy
115. transient scotomata
116. Exophthalmos
117. Dehydration
118. weight loss,

119. Leucocytosis
120. Headache
121. transient hyperglycemia
122. Hypercalcemia
123. Hyperparathyroidism
124. albuminuria,
125. excessive weight gain
126. edematous swelling of ankles
   or   wrists
127. metallic taste
128. dysgeusia/taste distortion,
129. salty taste
130. Thirst
131. swollen lips
132. tightness in chest
133. swollen and/or painful joints
134. Fever
135. polyarthralgia, and
136. dental caries.
137. nephrogenic diabetes
   insipidus,
138. hyperparathyroidism, and
139. hypothyroidism which persist
   after lithium discontinuation
140. A few reports have been
received of the development of
painful discoloration of fingers and
toes and coldness of the extremities
within one day of starting lithium
treatment.

Valproate (Depakote, Epilim)

Valproate is the second most effective medication for mood disorders.

It also comes with a heavy cost that includes but is not limited to:

Contraindicated in the presence of mitochondrial disorders and urea cycle disorders. Caution with mental retardation as mental retardation may be caused by urea cycle disorders and mitochondrial disorders.

1. Black box Warnings for:
2. Fatalities from hepatotoxicity
3. Risk of birth defects including spina bifida
4. Decreased IQ Following in utero Exposure
5. Fatal hemorrhagic pancreatitis
6. Suicidal behavior or ideation
7. Somnolence in the Elderly
8. valproate stimulates the replication of the HIV and CMV
9. Bleeding
10. hematopoietic disorders

27 of 64

11. Hyperammonemia
12. hyperammonemic encephalopathy
13. Hypothermia
14. Eosinophilia
15. Multiorgan hypersensitivity reaction Somnolence in the elderly
16. Most common adverse reactions
17. abdominal pain
18. Alopecia
19. Amblyopia
20. blurred vision
21. Amnesia
22. Anorexia
23. Asthenia
24. ataxia,
25. Bronchitis
26. Constipation
27. Depression
28. Diarrhea
29. Diplopia
30. dizziness,
31. Dyspepsia
32. Dyspnea
33. Ecchymosis
34. emotional lability
35. Fever
36. flu syndrome
37. Headache
38. increased appetite
39. Infection

40. Insomnia
41. Nausea
42. nervousness,
43. Nystagmus
44. peripheral edema
45. Pharyngitis
46. Rhinitis
47. Somnolence
48. Abnormal thinking
49. Thrombocytopenia
50. Tinnitus
51. Tremor
52. Vomiting
53. weight gain
54. weight loss
55. Dermatologic:
56. Hair texture changes,
57. hair color changes,
58. photosensitivity,
59. erythema multiforme,
60. toxic epidermal necrolysis,
61. nail and nail bed disorders
62. Stevens-Johnson syndrome.
63. Psychiatric:
64. Emotional upset
65. Psychosis
66. Aggression
67. psychomotor hyperactivity
68. hostility,
69. disturbance in attention

70. learning disorder
71. behavioral deterioration
72. Neurologic:
73. There have been several reports of acute or subacute cognitive decline
74. behavioral changes
75. Apathy
76. Irritability
77. cerebral pseudoatrophy on imaging
78. Musculoskeletal:
79. Fractures
80. decreased bone mineral density
81. Osteopenia
82. osteoporosis
83. Bone weakness.
84. Hematologic:
85. Relative lymphocytosis
86. Macrocytosis
87. Leucopenia
88. anemia including
89. Macrocytic anemia
90. bone marrow suppression
91. Pancytopenia
92. aplastic anemia,
93. Agranulocytosis
94. acute intermittent porphyria.
95. Endocrine:
96. Irregular menses
97. secondary amenorrhea
98. Hyperandrogenism

99. Hirsutism
100. Elevated testosterone level
101. breast enlargement
102. Galactorrhea
103. parotid gland swelling
104. polycystic ovary disease
105. decreased carnitine concentrations
106. Hyponatremia
107. hyperglycinemia, and
108. Inappropriate ADH secretion.
109. Fanconi's syndrome occurring chiefly in children inadequate reabsorption in the proximal renal tubules of the kidney excess amounts of glucose, bicarbonate, phosphates (phosphorus salts), uric acid, potassium, and certain amino acids being excreted in the urine.
110. Metabolism and nutrition:
111. Weight gain.
112. Reproductive:
113. Aspermia, azoospermia, decreased sperm count, decreased spermatozoa motility, male infertility, and abnormal spermatozoa morphology.
114. Genitourinary:
115. Enuresis and
116. urinary tract infection.

117.   Special Senses: Hearing loss.
118.   Other:
119.   Allergic reaction,
120.   anaphylaxis,
121.   developmental delay,
122.   bone pain,
123.   bradycardia, and
124.   cutaneous vasculitis.

Carbamazepine (Tegretol)

CYP 3A4 inhibitors inhibit Tegretol metabolism and can thus increase plasma carbamazepine levels. Drugs that have been shown, or would be expected, to increase plasma carbamazepine levels include but are not limited to: cimetidine, danazol, diltiazem, macrolides, erythromycin, troleandomycin, clarithromycin, fluoxetine, fluvoxamine, nefazodone, loratadine, terfenadine, isoniazid, niacinamide, nicotinamide, propoxyphene, azoles (e.g., ketaconazole, itraconazole, fluconazole), acetazolamide, verapamil, grapefruit juice, protease inhibitors, valproate.*

32 of 64

CYP 3A4 inducers can increase the rate of Tegretol metabolism. Drugs that have been shown, or that would be expected, to decrease plasma carbamazepine levels include but are not limited to: cisplatin, doxorubicin HCl, felbamate,† rifampin, phenobarbital, phenytoin, primidone, methsuximide, theophylline.

Tegretol induces hepatic CYP activity. Tegretol causes, or would be expected to cause, decreased levels of the following, but is not limited to the following: acetaminophen, alprazolam, dihydropyridine calcium channel blockers (e.g., felodipine), cyclosporine, corticosteroids (e.g., prednisolone, dexamethasone), clonazepam, clozapine, dicumarol, doxycycline, ethosuximide,haloperidol, itraconazole, lamotrigine, levothyroxine, methadone, methsuximide, midazolam, olanzapine, oral and other hormonal contraceptives, oxcarbazepine, phensuximide, phenytoin, praziquantel, protease inhibitors, risperidone, theophylline, tiagabine, topiramate, tramadol, tricyclic antidepressants (e.g., imipramine, amitriptyline, nortriptyline), valproate, warfarin, ziprasidone, zonisamide.

Black Box Warning

1. SERIOUS AND SOMETIMES FATAL DERMATOLOGIC REACTIONS, INCLUDING TOXIC EPIDERMAL NECROLYSIS (TEN) AND STEVENS-JOHNSON SYNDROME (SJS)
2. APLASTIC ANEMIA AND AGRANULOCYTOSIS
3. 50% of Asians with the HLA-B*1502 Allele will have Steven Johnson Syndrome and Toxic Epidermal Necrolysis (SJS/TEN) often with fatal outcomes. Asians with rash should stop Tegretol. Asians should be tested for the HLA-B*1502 Allele
4. Antiepileptic drugs (AEDs), including Tegretol, increase the risk of suicidal thoughts or behavior.
5. Tegretol has shown mild anticholinergic activity and can aggravate closed angle glaucoma.
6. Tegretol can cause birth defects and developmental delays including:
7. spina bifida

8. craniofacial defects
9. cardiovascular malformations
10. hypospadias
11. Developmental delays
12. Combining anticonvulsants increases the rates of birth defects;
13. AV heart block, including second and third degree block
14. hepatic failure
15. Multiorgan hypersensitivity reactions
16.

SYMPTOMS THAT INDICATE THE NEED TO STOP TEGRETOL INCLUDE:

17. Fever
18. sore throat
19. Rash
20. ulcers in the mouth
21. easy bruising
22. Lymphadenopathy
23. petechial or purpuric hemorrhage
24. Anorexia
25. Nausea
26. vomiting
27. Jaundice.

Other serious side effects include but are not limited to:
28. Hemopoietic System:
29. Aplastic anemia

30. Agranulocytosis
31. Pancytopenia
32. bone marrow depression
33. Thrombocytopenia
34. Leukopenia
35. Leukocytosis
36. Eosinophilia
37. acute intermittent porphyria
38. Skin
39. Toxic epidermal necrolysis (TEN) and Stevens-Johnson syndrome (SJS)
40. pruritic and erythematous rashes
41. Urticaria
42. photosensitivity reactions
43. alterations in skin pigmentation
44. exfoliative dermatitis
45. erythema multiforme and nodosum
46. Purpura
47. aggravation of disseminated lupus erythematosus
48. Alopecia
49. Diaphoresis
50. In certain cases, discontinuation of therapy may be necessary.
51. hirsutism
52. Cardiovascular System
53. Congestive heart failure
54. Edema
55. aggravation of hypertension

36 of 64

56. Hypotension
57. syncope and collapse
58. aggravation of coronary artery disease
59. arrhythmias
60. AV block
61. Thrombophlebitis
62. Thromboembolism
63. adenopathy
64. Lymphadenopathy
65. Myocardial infarction has been associated with other tricyclic compounds.
66. Liver: Abnormalities in liver function tests, cholestatic and hepatocellular jaundice, hepatitis; very rare cases of hepatic failure.
67. Pancreatic: Pancreatitis.
68. Respiratory System: Pulmonary hypersensitivity characterized by fever, dyspnea, pneumonitis, or pneumonia.
69. Genitourinary System: Urinary frequency, acute urinary retention, oliguria with elevated blood pressure, azotemia, renal failure, and impotence. Albuminuria, glycosuria, elevated BUN, and microscopic deposits in the urine have also been reported.

70. Nervous System:
71. Dizziness
72. Drowsiness
73. disturbances of coordination
74. Confusion
75. Headache
76. Fatigue
77. blurred vision
78. visual hallucinations
79. transient diplopia
80. oculomotor disturbances
81. Nystagmus
82. speech disturbances
83. abnormal involuntary movements
84. peripheral neuritis
85. Paresthesias
86. Depression
87. Agitation
88. Talkativeness
89. Tinnitus
90. hyperacusis.
91. Paralysis
92. symptoms of cerebral arterial insufficiency
93. neuroleptic malignant syndrome
94. Digestive System:
95. Nausea
96. Vomiting
97. gastric distress
98. abdominal pain

99.   Diarrhea
100.   Constipation
101.   Anorexia
102.   dryness of the mouth and
       pharynx
103.   glossitis
104.   Stomatitis
105.   Eyes:
106.   punctate cortical lens
       opacities
107.   Conjunctivitis
108.   Musculoskeletal System:
109.   Aching joints and muscles
110.   leg cramps
111.   Metabolism
112.   Fever and chills
113.   Inappropriate antidiuretic
       hormone (ADH)
114.   water intoxication
115.   decreased serum
       sodium(hyponatremia)
116.   Confusion
117.   Decreased levels of plasma
       calcium
118.   Multiorgan hypersensitivity
reactions fever, skin rashes,
vasculitis, lymphadenopathy,
disorders mimicking lymphoma,
arthralgia, leukopenia, eosinophilia,
hepatosplenomegaly and abnormal

39 of 64

liver function tests affecting the
liver, skin, immune system, lungs,
kidneys, pancreas, myocardium, and
colon may be affected
119.   lupus erythematosus-like
         syndrome
120.   elevated levels of cholesterol,
HDL cholesterol, and triglycerides
in patients taking anticonvulsants
121.   aseptic meningitis,
accompanied by myoclonus and
peripheral eosinophilia

Lamotrigine (Lamictal) Adverse effectis
include, but are not limited to the
following:

BLACK BOX WARNING:
Stevens-Johnson syndrome and toxic
epidermal necrolysis, and/or rash-related
death
Increased risk when combined with
valproate; exceeding recommended
initial dose of LAMICTAL; exceeding
recommended dose escalation for
LAMICTAL.
LAMICTAL should be discontinued at the
first sign of rash, unless the rash is clearly
not drug related.

ADDITIONAL WARNINGS:
1. Blood dyscrasias
2. Neutropenia
3. Thrombocytopenia
4. Pancytopenia
5. Suicidal behavior and ideation
6. Aseptic meningitis Symptoms include headache, fever, nausea, vomiting, and nuchal rigidity. Rash, photophobia, myalgia, chills, altered consciousness, and somnolence were also noted in some cases.

Most Common Adverse Reactions:
Epilepsy
Most common adverse reactions (incidence ≥10%) in adults were
1. Dizziness
2. Headache
3. Diplopia
4. Ataxia
5. Nausea
6. blurred vision,
7. Somnolence
8. Rhinitis
9. Pharyngitis
10. rash.

Bipolar disorder: Most common adverse reactions (incidence >5%
1. Nausea
2. Insomnia
3. Somnolence
4. back pain
5. Fatigue
6. Rash
7. Rhinitis
8. abdominal pain
9. Xerostomia

Less Common Side effects include:
1. lamotrigine binds to melanin and over time may cause toxicity
2. Body as a whole
3. Headache
4. Flu syndrome
5. Fever
6. Abdominal pain
7. Neck pain
8. Digestive Nausea
9. Vomiting
10. Diarrhea
11. Dyspepsia
12. Constipation
13. Anorexia
14. Musculoskeletal
15. Arthralgia
16. Nervous

42 of 64

17. Dizziness
18. Ataxia
19. Somnolence
20. Incoordination
21. Insomnia
22. Tremor
23. Depression
24. Anxiety
25. Convulsion
26. Irritability
27. Speech disorder
28. Concentration disturbance
29. Respiratory
30. Rhinitis
31. Pharyngitis
32. Cough increased
33. Skin and appendages
34. Rash
35. Pruritus
36. Special senses
37. Diplopia
38. Blurred vision
39. Vision abnormality
40. Urogenital Female patients only
41. Dysmenorrhea
42. Vaginitis
43. Amenorrhea

44. Adverse reactions that occurred with a frequency of less than 5% and greater than 1% of patients
45. receiving LAMICTAL and numerically more frequent than placebo were:
46. General:
47. Fever
48. neck pain
49. Cardiovascular
50. Migraine
51. Digestive
52. Flatulence
53. Metabolic and Nutritional:
54. Weight gain
55. Edema
56. Musculoskeletal
57. Arthralgia
58. Myalgia
59. Nervous System:
60. Amnesia
61. Depression
62. Agitation
63. emotional lability
64. Dyspraxia
65. abnormal thoughts
66. dream abnormality
67. Hypoesthesia

68. Respiratory
69. Sinusitis
70. Urogenital
71. Urinary frequency
72. Adverse Reactions Following Abrupt Discontinuation:
73. increase in the incidence, severity, or type of adverse reactions in patients with bipolar disorder after abruptly terminating therapy with LAMICTAL.
74. seizures
75. mania
76. hypomania
77. mixed mood episodes
78. Postmarketing Experience
79. Blood and Lymphatic
80. Agranulocytosis
81. hemolytic anemia
82. lymphadenopathy
83. . Gastrointestinal
84. Esophagitis
85. Hepatobiliary Tract and Pancreas
86. Pancreatitis
87. Immunologic
88. Lupus-like reaction
89. Vasculitis
90. Lower Respiratory

91. Apnea
92. Musculoskeletal
93. Rhabdomyolysis
94. Nervous System
95. Aggression
96. exacerbation of Parkinsonian symptoms
97. Non-site Specific P
98. progressive immunosuppression.

Anorexia: starvation. Psychiatric treatment often fails and there are quite a few newspaper articles of rich and famous people dying from anorexia nervosa despite multiple hospital admissions and extensive psychiatric treatments.

Pathological Gambling: this may result in loss of business, home and family.

Addictions to Drugs and Alcohol: this may result in loss of business, home, family and health.

Factitious Disorder: the need to have a physical or mental illness strong enough to feign physical or mental illness.

Munchhausen Disorder: an extreme form of factitious disorder whereby the patient goes from doctor to doctor until efforts secure a diagnosis and treatment with frequent doctor and emergency room visits. The focus appears to be the need to have extensive time with a medical doctor.

Munchhausen by Proxy: this involves the need to have a child or other dependent with a diagnosis of a physical or mental illness with frequent office and emergency room visits. Again, the focus appears to be the need to have extensive time with medical doctor.

Malingering. The malingerer fakes mental illness to secure disability benefits, time off from work, not guilty by insanity, or money in a civil suit. This is not a mental illness and there is no effective treatment for criminal behavior.

Having taken a superficial look at the landscape of mental health and mental illness, let's look at the individual in the office.

The individual should identify symptoms that are on the table for treatment.

The individual should rate the symptoms on a scale of 0 to 10, 0 being none to 10 the worst ever experienced that have been a recent problem.

The patient should state the frequency, duration, and impaired function of symptoms over the course of the prior month. The patient should then commit to keeping a diary of the symptoms and impaired function during treatment.

The patient should initially try controlling the symptoms with exercise to reduce anxiety and depression, meditation to reduce anxiety and depression and to increase focus and attention, sleep hygiene to improve sleep, dietary hygiene to optimize weight and physical health, breathing exercises to control anxiety, social hygiene to improve interpersonal relationships and reduce stress, and psychotherapy to target symptoms of mental illness.

At each appointment the patient should review the diary.

If the above interventions fail, then the patient should consider psychotropic medications.

The risks and benefits should be reviewed, and the patient should commit to a trial of four to eight weeks on each medication before trying a second medication.

If there are allergic or other serious adverse effects of the medication the patient should stop the medication, go to an emergency room and then consult with the psychiatrist regarding another medication trial.

I suggest the reader review, Meditation Medications and Your First Psychiatric Consultation, by William R. Yee M.D., JD and The Best Practice Is The Lowest Effective Dose, Your Third Psychiatric Consultation Copyright Applied for 11/03/2019, All rights reserved, William R. Yee M.D., J.D.

The reader should understand that the mechanism of action of psychotropic medications are not understood because the brain has 100 billion neurons and 100 trillion synapses connecting the 100 billion neurons. The brain is too complex to be understood at this time. Therefore, mental health and mental illness are not understood. Therefore, the ways that medications work on mental illness are not understood.

There is a dispute as to whether psychotropic medications are effective and better than placeboes.

Because there are no cures, the goal is a "functional recovery."

Analysis of medical records in socialized medicine documents the fact that the functional recovery of psychosis or schizophrenia is doubled when the medication is stopped after six months,

There are assessments of medication trials that result in medications only achieving a 2% benefit.

There are assessments of antidepressant trials that indicate that antidepressants are no better than placebo.

There is also research that indicate that some patients benefit from psychotropic medications.

Since I am a psychiatrist and the insurance industry and clinics confine my practice to prescribing medications, I advise patients that I will let them try one medication at a time until they find a medication that works for them or until they decide that it is not worth taking medications at all.

At this point we list all the symptoms that the patient wants resolved and the patient rates the range of severity of the symptom over the past month and the amount of disability.

Symptom are rated at 0 for none to 10 the worst experienced by the patient during the patient's lifetime.

It is often worthwhile to state the circumstances at the time the symptom was a ten.

The diary should record circumstances.

In addition to rating the severity, the duration and frequency of symptoms should be recorded.

Disability 0 none to 10 complete disability.

Anxiety   0 1 2 3 4 5 6 7 8 9 10
Disability   0 1 2 3 4 5 6 7 8 9 10
Frequency   ____ times a day week
month
Duration   ___ to ___   Hours
Minutes
Depression   0 1 2 3 4 5 6 7 8 9 10
Disability   0 1 2 3 4 5 6 7 8 9 10
Frequency   ____ times a day week
month
Duration   ___ to ___   Hours
Minutes
Hallucinations 0 1 2 3 4 5 6 7 8 9 10
Disability   0 1 2 3 4 5 6 7 8 9 10
Frequency   ____ times a day week
month
Duration   ___ to ___   Hours
Minutes Delusions   0 1 2 3 4 5 6 7 8 9
10
Disability   0 1 2 3 4 5 6 7 8 9 10
Frequency   ____ times a day week
month

Duration	__ to __	Hours

Minutes

Paranoia	0 1 2 3 4 5 6 7 8 9 10
Disability	0 1 2 3 4 5 6 7 8 9 10
Frequency	____ times a day week

month

Duration	__ to __	Hours

Minutes

Sleep	__Hours per night
	__ Interruptions per night
Appetite	Increased Decreased Weight

The symptoms can be listed on a sheet of paper on columns 1 to 31 for the days of the month

This should be brought into each appointment for review and to modify treatment over time.

1 Anxiety   0 1 2 3 4 5 6 7 8 9 10 Disability
0 1 2 3 4 5 6 7 8 9 10
Frequency __ times a day week month
Duration __ Hours Minutes
2 Anxiety   0 1 2 3 4 5 6 7 8 9 10 Disability
0 1 2 3 4 5 6 7 8 9 10
Frequency __ times a day week month
Duration __ Hours Minutes
3 Anxiety   0 1 2 3 4 5 6 7 8 9 10
53 of 64

Disability 0 1 2 3 4 5 6 7 8 9 10
Frequency __ times a day week month
Duration __ Hours Minutes

30 Anxiety   0 1 2 3 4 5 6 7 8 9 10 Disability
0 1 2 3 4 5 6 7 8 9 10
Frequency __ times a day week month
Duration __ Hours Minutes
31 Anxiety   0 1 2 3 4 5 6 7 8 9 10
Disability 0 1 2 3 4 5 6 7 8 9 10
Frequency __ times a day week month
Duration __ Hours Minutes

The patient can write notes in the
margins regarding precipitating and
changing circumstances.

This can be entered into the patient
record to document patient participation
and progression of symptoms in response
to treatment.

The choice of medications is important.

By the time the primary physician has
referred the patient to the psychiatrist
the use of addicting medications is no
longer an option.

54 of 64

Ambien is only useful for a week or two and Xanax can cause withdrawal seizures with five days of exposure.
The reader should review Michael Jackson's experience with sleeping pills and addicting medications to understand the result of long-term use of addicting medications.

SSRI's and SNRI's are used for depression, anxiety and panic attacks. This is because anxiety and depression often occur together, and the underlying pathology of depression and anxiety are in part shared both in the brain and in the environmental stresses of life experience.
Selective serotonin reuptake inhibitors (SSRIs)
Citalopram (Celexa)
Escitalopram (Lexapro)
Fluoxetine (Prozac)
Fluvoxamine (Luvox)
Paroxetine (Paxil)
Sertraline (Zoloft)
SNRIs
desvenlafaxine (Pristiq)
duloxetine (Cymbalta)
levomilnacipran (Fetzima)
venlafaxine (Effexor)

There is no antidepressant that is so superior to the rest that it would be malpractice not to start with that medication.

The antidepressants are about equally effective and differ primarily in side effects.

I usually start with Escitalopram because it has the least side effects and is most tolerated antidepressant on average.

You need to treat seven depressed or anxious patients to find one that responds to Lexapro. With each medication trial after Lexapro that number gets larger.

The definition of benefit was a 50% reduction of symptoms. You treat seven patients before you find one patient that has a 50% reduction of symptoms.

The number to treat to harm for antidepressants is larger than the number to treat for benefit. You treat more than seven patients before you find one patient that is harmed by the medication.

56 of 64

The definition if harm is a side effect severe enough for the patient to stop taking the medication.

Typical antipsychotics include:
1. Haldol (haloperidol)
2. Loxitane (loxapine)
3. Mellaril (thioridazine)
4. Moban (molindone)
5. Navane (thiothixene)
6. Prolixin (fluphenazine)
7. Serentil (mesoridazine)
8. Stelazine (trifluoperazine)
9. Trilafon (perphenazine)
10. Thorazine (chlorpromazine)

Antipsychotics are generally equally effective and the choice is generally made upon side effects.

Perphanzine has been found to be the most cost effective and is often a first choice.

I generally offer chlorpromazine first because it is also effective for bipolar disorder, anxiety, aggression, insomnia and calms the patient down more quickly and effectively than other antipsychotic medications.

I have been treating mental illness since 1972 and have more experience with chlorpromazine than most younger psychiatrists.

That said, it remains the patient's choice.

Atypical antipsychotics include:
1. Abilify (aripiprazole)
2. Clozaril (clozapine)
3. Geodon (ziprasidone)
4. Risperdal (risperidone)
5. Seroquel (quetiapine)
6. Zyprexa (olanzapine)

Atypical antipsychotics in general are no better than typical antipsychotics.

All antipsychotics have a black box warning for death in the elderly with dementia.

The elderly in general have a lower physiologic reserve than the young. The elderly die at higher rates than the young when exposed to any stressor. There is no scientific basis for stating that the elderly without dementia are at less risk of death from antipsycotics than the elderly with dementia.

58 of 64

That said, the older a patient is, the more important it is to wean him off antipsychotic medications.

Although Clozaril has achieved some notoriety as the, "Gold Standard," for the treatment of psychosis, it comes with a heavy price in morbidity and mortality, i.e. suffering and death.

Some of the literature disputes the putative superiority of Clozaril/Clozapine.

Part of its success may be based upon the extra time spent with the patient monitoring for lethal side effects. It is known that time spent with mental health professionals is associated with a reduction of symptoms.

Part of its success may be based upon a combination of placebo effect and cognitive dissonance. It is hard to justify the risk of death without benefit. It is easier to justify the risk of death with a benefit, ergo a benefit.

The high price of clozaril includes, but is not limited to the following:

Black box warnings for:
Seizures;
Myocarditis manifesting with
unexplained fatigue, dyspnea, tachypnea,
fever, chest pain, palpitations, other signs
or symptoms of heart failure, or
electrocardiographic findings such as ST-
T wave abnormalities or arrhythmias,
exertional dyspnea, fatigue, orthopnea,
paroxysmal nocturnal dyspnea, and
peripheral edema ;
Orthostatic Hypotension;
Syncope;
Respiratory Arrest;
Cardiac Arrest;
Additional Serious Side Effects include:
but are not limited to:
Agranulocytosis that requires weekly
blood testing for ANC;
Eosinophilia;
Hyperglycemia and Diabetes Mellitus:
Neuroleptic Malignant Syndrome (NMS)
Tardive Dyskinesia
Pulmonary Embolism;
Hepatitis;
Anticholinergic Toxicity;
Interference with Cognitive and Motor
Performance;
Withdrawal symptoms include:
CNS, primarily drowsiness/sedation,

seizures, dizziness/syncope;
cardiovascular, primarily tachycardia,
hypotension and ECG changes;
gastrointestinal, primarily nausea
Dystonia;
Side Effects by system include:
Central Nervous System
Drowsiness/Sedation
Dizziness/Vertigo
Headache
Tremor
Syncope
Disturbed Sleep/Nightmares
Restlessness
Hypokinesia/Akinesia
Agitation
Seizures (convulsions)
Rigidity
Akathisia
Confusion
Fatigue
Insomnia
Hyperkinesia
Weakness
Lethargy
Ataxia
Slurred Speech
Depression
Epileptiform Movements/Myoclonic Jerks
Anxiety

Cardiovascular
Tachycardia
Hypotension
Hypertension
Chest Pain/Angina
ECG Change/Cardiac Abnormality
Gastrointestinal
Constipation
Nausea
Abdominal Discomfort/Heartburn
Nausea/Vomiting
Vomiting
Diarrhea
Liver test Abnormality
Anorexia
Urogenital
Urinary Abnormalities
Incontinence
Abnormal Ejaculation
Urinary Urgency/Frequency
Urinary Retention
Autonomic Nervous System
Salivation
Sweating
Dry Mouth
Visual Disturbances
Integumentary (Skin)
Rash
Musculoskeletal
Muscle Weakness

Pain (Back, Neck, Legs)
Muscle Spasm
Muscle Pain, Ache
Respiratory
Throat Discomfort
Dyspnea, Shortness of Breath
Nasal Congestion
Hemic/Lymphatic
Leukopenia/Decreased WBC/Neutropenia
Agranulocytosis
Eosinophilia
Miscellaneous
Fever
Weight Gain
Tongue Numb/Sore

The side effects of Clozaril also occur with other antipsychotic medications, but with less severity and less frequency.

The FDA Label for the chosen medication should be reviewed before taking the medication. Also, after release for commercial sale, new information will appear on the internet before it is included in later iterations of the original FDA label.

I tell the patient that I will prescribe one medication at time until the patient finds
63 of 64

a medication that works well enough for the patient to want to stay on that medication.

At some point the treatment should be terminated as a success or a failure with a referral for alternative treatment or a second opinion.
At some point this commentary must end.
Thank you for your time and attention.
This introduction will soon be obsolete.
I hope that archeologists will find it useful in the distant future.

William R. Yee M.D., J.D.

"Preexisting text," includes names of mental illnesses, symptoms of mental illnesses, FDA Labels and the contents of FDA labels cited in the text.

My copyright claim is a clam to the "original text," which is my personal experiences as described in the text above and my commentary on the names of mental illnesses, symptoms of mental illnesses, FDA Labels and the contents of FDA labels cited in the text cited.